Weight Loss for Women

Seventeen Day Diet

By Cathy Wilson
Copyright © 2014

Income Disclaimer

This book contains business strategies, marketing methods and other business advice that, regardless of my own results and experience, may not produce the same results (or any results) for you. I make absolutely no guarantee, expressed or implied, that by following the advice below you will make any money or improve current profits, as there are several factors and variables that come into play regarding any given business.

Primarily, results will depend on the nature of the product or business model, the conditions of the marketplace, the experience of the individual, and situations and elements that are beyond your control.

As with any business endeavor, you assume all risk related to investment and money based on your own discretion and at your own potential expense.

Liability Disclaimer

By reading this book, you assume all risks associated with using the advice given below, with a full understanding that you, solely, are responsible for anything that may occur as a result of putting this information into action in any way, and regardless of your interpretation of the advice.

You further agree that our company cannot be held responsible in any way for the success or failure of your business as a result of the information presented in this book. It is your responsibility to conduct your own due diligence regarding the safe and successful operation of your business if you intend to apply any of our information in any way to your business operations.

Terms of Use

You are given a non-transferable, "personal use" license to this book. You cannot distribute it or share it with other individuals.

Also, there are no resale rights or private label rights granted when purchasing this book. In other words, it's for your own personal use only.

Weight Loss for Women

Seventeen Day Diet

By Cathy Wilson

Thank you for downloading my book! I appreciate it and I worked hard researching and writing to provide you with the best book possible. Unfortunately, I'm not a famous author yet, and I don't have at my disposal, a qualified team of writers, researchers, editors, marketers, etc., to put my book on the map. I do it all myself, with the exception of the cover. And I just want to remind you that I am not perfect and neither is this book. I am a very good writer always looking to improve, and welcome any constructive criticisms you have to help me deliver bigger and better each time.

An open mind thirsting for new knowledge is a beautiful thing.

If you gain just one piece of useful information, or even just smile once or twice, then I am content. Time to open your mind, enjoy, and look for what you can gain from my book! Thank you again, and at the end of the book, you will find a link to my website and all my other books offering solutions to better your health and life.

Happy reading!

Table of Contents

Introduction

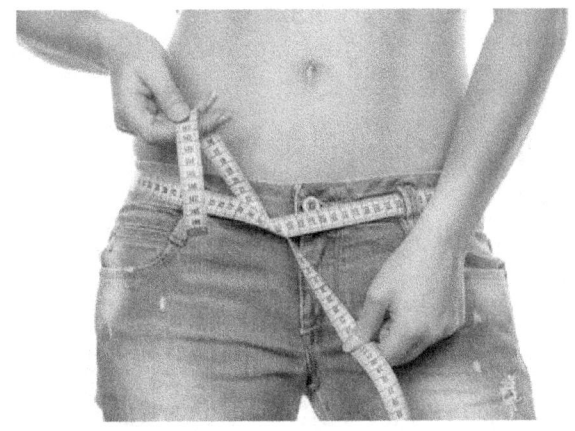

If you want to sum this diet up, it's all about LOSING WEIGHT FAST.

Is this diet perfect? Nope. Am I perfect? Not even close. Is this book going to help you blast fat fast, and improve your health immensely? YES! YES! YES! It's all about perspective, as with everything in life. YOU choose the bits and pieces from all the information you ingest, that can be used to make your life better. There's only good in that, because you deserve to be healthy, happy, and inspired for more.

I am a health and nutrition expert, with over 20 years experience, and numerous health and wellness books in publication. I have always learned by doing, and now look forward to passing this wealth of information onto you. If you gain at least one useful piece of knowledge you can apply to positively affect your life, then I've made this book worth my while.
How does the 17 Day Diet work?

It's done sensibly using your natural body mechanics, in combination with how your systems work internally; considering your tolerances and preferences, what you enjoy, and what you can't stand. Never forgetting there are some factors that are absolute. If you want to lose weight and keep it off, you are going to have to . . .

* **Make healthier food choices**
* **Eat less calories than your body expends**
* **Fit physical activity into things you enjoy doing**

As with each and every diet strategy out there, theories or factors, are in place to deliver you to your desired weight loss within a specific time frame. If you know when to expect weight loss before you begin, it's perceived as success. The 17 Day Diet sets you up for success. If you've got 17 days to commit to following this plan, you WILL lose fat and get one step closer to a healthier and happier you.

Time to open your mind and turn on your determination so we can get started!

17 Day Diet Basics

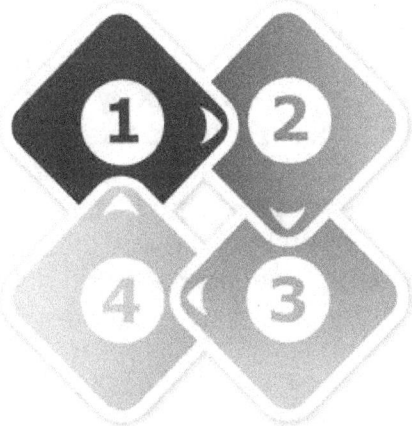

This scientific based diet is broken down into 4 x 17 day cycles, so it easier to digest. Cleaning your house one room at a time is manageable. Trying to clean it spic and span in one shot is depressing and freaking crazy! While reading through this well-balanced and logical diet, keep in mind perspective. Take the information that makes sense to you. Open your mind to absorb and learn new tactics and strategies, to help improve your health, and always look at the big picture. It's not about being right or wrong here, but if you choose, the 17 Day Diet WILL fit. The four main cycles in this diet are:

ACCELERATE
ACTIVATE
ACHIEVE

ARRIVE

The idea behind this lifestyle change is a common-sense approach, teaching your body how to run optimally with a few key, and repetitive steps. First, is to get rid of all the toxins and harmful chemicals in your body built up over time. Science says your body is not made to process anything but ALL NATURAL foods, which means sweet and tasty processed foods with zero nutrition and mountains of fat, have no place to go. Your body can't deal with chemicals, preservatives, and bad fats, particularly in the oceanic amounts we eat them. Sodas, burgers, fries, chips, chocolate bars, cakes and pastries, poison your body, interfering with each and every internal system. Stealing energy, triggering sickness and disease, and making your life very depressing, often ending it prematurely.

Purging your system of this reservoir of poison makes sense.

Slowly, with this practical eating style, you add healthy and nutritious foods back into your system. Trying to show your body it can trust you, and you that you WILL feed it premium fuel. The benefits are crazy fast weight loss, energy levels shooting up, minor ailments start to dissipate, chronic conditions take a turn for the better, and preventative measures are in place to stay far away from serious disease. You also benefit your mental by looking and feeling better, which makes all the difference in the world. Measures are put into place to set you up for maintaining your weight loss, and smart and energetic eating patterns, which is important if you really do care about you.

With this diet, regular physical exercise is essential to make your results stick. It's not about exercising strenuously by any means, rather implementing daily physical activity into your schedule to help boost your metabolism and make your body work more effectively for you. With regular exercise your internal systems and your mental will both run more effectively.

This is NOT a cyclical fad diet full of broken promises and inevitably broken scales. In basic, the 17 Day Diet is a concept of losing fat fast, gaining energy, and deterring disease, that is sensible and effective, a lifestyle move that will stick IF you are willing to work for it. Habits are hard to break but this one is just too important to ignore. You matter.

My Thoughts . . .
It doesn't matter how you look at it. If you don't truly "want" to lose weight and get healthy, then please don't waste your time. When you are ready, the 17 Day Diet will be ready and waiting to propel you to your weight loss goals fast.
This diet is all about sensible eating, diversity, control and reward, and implementing exercise regularly in a manageable and positive light. Talk about a plan destined to succeed!

Powerful Benefits of Weight Loss

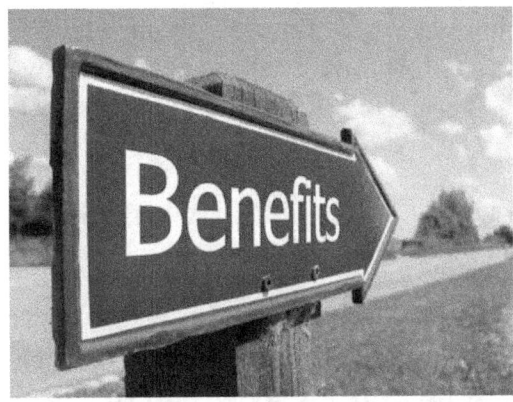

It's essentially a universal fact that everyone on the face of this earth would like to drop at least a few pounds. Even those stick-pin models without an ounce of body fat want to get thinner! It's crazy, but true.

For most of us, losing weight is a good thing. It's not just about that "feel good" feeling you get when you have to do your belt a notch tighter, or go shopping for a new dress because your old one just doesn't hug your curves anymore. Your body was programmed with what I call a "weight meter." This meter is set at your "ideal" weight. The point in which your body feels it functions optimally. Of course this is different for each of us.

What happens over time through external factors, is we muck the safety mechanism up. Depriving ourselves of calories and sleep. Then we overload it with fats and junk food. Back and forth like a ping pong ball causes our me-ter to reset at an unhealthy weight, which naturally makes it even harder for us to drop fat even when we want to. We cause the negative interference.

Lucky for us we CAN lower our weight and reset our internal weight meter at a healthier weight, if we commit to sensibly losing the weight and keep it off for at least 6 months. This is how long it takes for your body to trust you enough to believe you are finally going to keep your weight where it should, healthy and true.

Truth is, if I was your body I wouldn't trust you either - would you?
Here are a few more benefits from dropping fat and keeping it off!

* **Lengthens Life** -Studies show, people that suffer from an obesity-related disease such as diabetes, have an increased length of life by losing weight and improved quality too.

* **Found Money** - By cutting out chips, cakes, and expensive fast foods to lose weight, you're going to find lots and lots of money. Even if you just removed one small bag of chips, one chocolate bar, and one can of soda per week, which could save you about $144 per year!

* **Better Sex** - Experts agree that losing weight makes you more confident in your appearance and more likely to "feel" sexy. For men, obesity lowers testosterone levels, and decreasing sex drive. Studies show, by losing fat, testosterone levels jump drastically, and that's all good between the sheets.

* **Bring Forth the Energizer Bunny!** - Losing weight will literally take the weight of the world off your shoulders. Fat weighs you down physically and mentally. With the 17 Day Diet you will lose weight, gaining energy and pos-

itive life perspective throughout the process. The more fat that you lose, the more positives you gain.

Other Benefits include . . .
* Decreased cholesterol levels
* Lower blood pressure
* Better mobility and agility
* Increased respiratory function
* Less annoying aches and pains
* Better sleep
* More alert
* Increased productivity
* Better work relations
* Improved memory and cognitive capacity
* Lower blood sugar levels
* Decreased risk of diabetes, cardiovascular, cancers, and other serious illness
* Less risk for depression and anxiety
* Increase in optimism
* Less wear and tear on skeletal system
* Improvement in circulation, and internal system function
* Improved self-confidence, and positive life direction
* Able to handle stress better

According to experts, over SIXTY PERCENT of Americans are overweight or obese. That number scares the living crap out of me. Weight is something people can control. Don't you think it's about time we started taking action? So much devastation, struggling and destruction, goes hand-in-hand with obesity. The 17 Day Diet is a logical and sustainable option to turn your world right side up! It's up to YOU to pry your brain open to it.

My Thoughts . . .
Life is what you make it. Are you a positive or pessimistic person? I have no use for negativity, because it's magnetic in nature, pulling you in and stomping on your head

19

in the blink of an eye. By making the choice to commit to changing your life for the better, to lose fat and keep it off, while gaining all sorts of other vital life benefits, you will experience just how fantastic life is.

The 17 Day Diet will help you establish new positive life perspective, and make every single life challenge that much better for you. If you like to smile and feel good about yourself and life, or at least want to try, the 17 Day Diet has your name written all over it. Take from it the healthy nutrition concepts that work, and apply to your master health plan.

Phase 1 - Accelerate (Day 1-17)

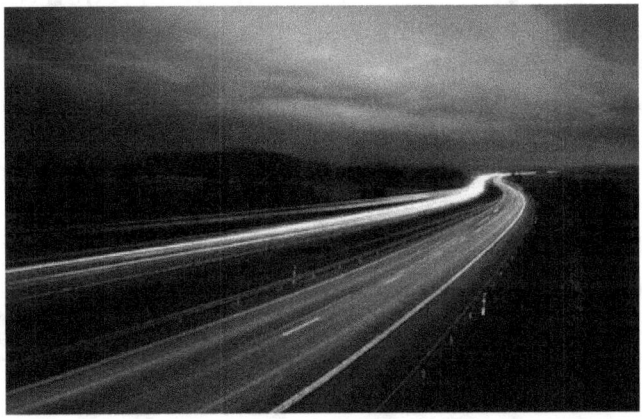

This first phase has the cards stacked against you, simply because it's different. People DO NOT like change, and find comfort in habit. Understand you will need to change your way of eating, and perspective in exercising, if you expect results. Wrap your head around this, and you are definitely moving in the right direction.

The concept here is to lower your daily caloric intake down to around 1200 calories per day, shocking your system. Many people lose up to 15 pounds in this phase, because of the extreme change to your system. You are underfeeding your body, still within the healthy range, while gaining the trust and support of your body by fueling your system only with the essential vitamins and minerals it requires to function optimally. It's not going to be stressed anymore trying to purge your system of all the excess fats and toxins it's used to.
A positive step.

Did you know there is such a thing as eating too little? If you don't give your body enough energy to at least match the energy demands you place on it, you will force your body to systematically shut down. Your internal systems will flip into "starvation mode," because that's exactly what you are doing. This means any morsel of food you do eat is going to be stored as fat because your body doesn't trust you.

Your body doesn't know when you are going to feed it again, so it is going to instinctively lower your metabolism, burn less calories, and try to use as little energy as possible for your body function. For bonus points, you're going to feel like crap too. By not fueling your body adequately, you are forcing it to fight you in losing weight.

What is the bottom line? You've GOT to eat to lose weight!

With the 17 Day Diet you are restricting calories in this phase, but you aren't going so low that your body fights you with the weight loss battle. You are also cleverly setting yourself up for reward with this phase.

Understanding your psychosomatic, or how your perceive things, are just as important as the actions you're taking. How you think and feel is incredibly vital.

This diet phase has a built-in motivator to keep you going; a few to be more precise. The first, is that you are going to see fast weight loss results, and that will make you want more. Also, you KNOW that in a few days you will be rewarded with more fuel for your body. You will be encouraged to eat more, and this in itself is extremely motivational.

Who doesn't want to eat more? The difference will be what you eat, when, and how much? It's important you stay strong here, because the last thing you want is to get lazy, feel defeated, and fall back into the deadly trap of your "olden day" eating patterns.

Cycle 1 hydrates, cleanses, removes toxins and un-healthy carb traces from your physical system, while triggering the burning of fat, and encouraging memory loss when it comes to unhealthy eating.

Exercising is critical with any long-term weight loss pro-gram. The 17 Day Diet plan sets you up for at least 17 minutes a day during both this first cycle and the next one. This exercising is very mild and can consist or just walking if you like. In the later cycles this strategy will shift gears to intense.

Sample Foods Cycle One
The last thing we want to do here is make this lifestyle change confusing or difficult. In this cycle you're encour-aged to eat lots of lean protein; including chicken, beef, eggs, and fish. Add to that lots of healthy fibrous, and nu-tritionally dense vegetables to start.

Low-fat, no sugar, and next to zero starchy carbs like white pasta, white bread and white rice are important. With cycle 1 you should consume a minimum of 2 probi-otics each day, with fresh fruits lowest in sugar; plums, berries and apples, are examples.

Carbohydrate intake throughout this cycle comes from low sugar fruits and needs to be munched before two o'clock each day. For hydration, and a boost to cleaning out your systems by drinking at least 8 ounces of warm lemon water upon waking, jumpstarting your digestive tract. Enjoying green tea at every meal is going to boost your metabolic process, while drinking 8 ounces of crystal clear water each day is going to make certain your fluids are running clear and your energy is optimal.

Vegetables to Cleanse
Asparagus, artichoke
Bell peppers, Brussels sprouts, broccoli
Celery, cauliflower, cabbage, carrots, cauliflower
Green beans, and leafy green vegetables, garlic
Leeks, lettuce, kale
Onions, mushrooms, and parsley
Spinach, scallions, tomatoes, and watercress

Fruit- Fibrous - 2 portions each day
All berries, apples, oranges, grapefruit
Pears, plums, peaches, nectarines, red grapes

Lean Protein
Chicken, skinless
Salmon, canned, broiled, grilled, baked
Tuna fish, water version
Lean turkey, skinless
Eggs; 2 per serving, or 4 egg whites
Sole, catfish, flounder, fresh lake perch, or bass

Probiotics - 2 portions each day
Sugar-free yogurt - 1 portion
Sauerkraut - 1/2 cup per serving
Acidophilous milk - 1 cup per serving
Kefir - 1 cup per serving
Yakult - 1 cup per serving

Fats 1-2 tbsp each day
Flaxseed or olive oil

Condiments - sparingly

Salsa, ketchup, sugar-free jams and jellies, low-fat sour cream, fat-free salad dressing, salt, pepper, mustard, spices, herbs, fat-free cheese, cooking spray, lite soy sauce

Vegan Adjustments
1/2 cup tofu
2 vegetarian black bean burgers
1/2 cup beans or lentils
2 veggie sausage links
Up to 4 oz vegan cheese
2 scoops vegan rice protein powder
DAIRY SUBSTITUTIONS - 1 portion is one cup non-sweet soy, almond, or rice milk. For yogurt use soy version

Sample Meals - 1200 calories per day

Day One

Breakfast
Hot lemon water
1/2 sugar-free yogurt
1 cup fresh berries
Green tea
Water

Lunch
Grilled chicken breast with two cups Romaine lettuce with tomatoes, carrots, celery and drizzle of low-fat salad dressing
Pear, or apple sliced
Green tea
Water

Dinner
1 serving grilled salmon (4-6oz)

2 cups steamed veggies (asparagus, red, yellow and orange peppers)
Green Tea
Water

Snacks
1 cup carrots/celery
1/2 cup sugar-free yogurt
Day Two

Breakfast
Warm lemon water
2 boiled eggs
1 cup fresh fruit - oranges, grapefruit, red grapes
Green Tea
Water

Lunch
Grilled lean turkey breast
Mixed vegetables - broccoli, eggplant, artichoke
1 serving low-fat yogurt
Apple sliced
Green Tea
Water

Dinner
Can of tuna in water
2 cups spinach, carrots, radishes, celery, cucumber, drizzle low-fat salad dressing
Green Tea
Water

Snacks
1 cup mixed veggies
1/2 low-fat yogurt with 1/4 fresh berries
The idea here is to ensure you mix and match these healthy foods as you see fit. Gear it towards your prefer-

ences and tolerances, and stick with the plan. During this first cycle you need to make huge adjustments in your eating. Lowering your daily caloric intake to 1200, boosting your fluid intake tremendously, and making sure you stick to the foods on the list, at least to start. Keep pace with this first eating cycle, include exercising for at least 17 minutes each day, and you will be cleansed, energized, and ready mentally and physically for cycle 2!

Phase 2 - Activate (Day 18-34)

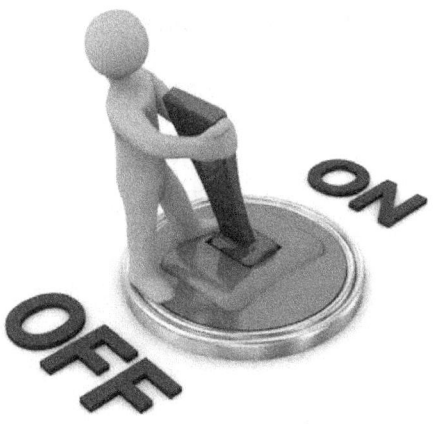

In this phase, you are re-activating your system, or rather starting it back up on a fresh new path. The food plan integrates a few more calories than Cycle 1 did. Think of it as your system being rewarded positively. Here, you are keeping your metabolic process on its toes, thinking and guessing, as to what you're going to throw at it next. This thought process maximizes the energy utilized, which gets you fat loss results fast.

This switch in gears also helps to starve off boredom, the number one cause of diet failure today. Although more than the previous phase, the calorie intake is still low enough to continue on the path of weight loss, losing another 5-8 pounds on average with Phase 2. It's better than a sharp stick in the eye for sure!

During this phase, you're going to need to add 2 servings of natural starches every other day, eaten before 2 pm.

Phase 2 lasts from day 18 to 34. Making sure you continue to focus on maximizing your nutrients, and minimizing calories, with healthy lean food choices, that give your body the nutrients critical for optimal function. A learning process always, and don't forget if you fall off the horse, recognize what you're doing, and get your butt back up there pronto - no worries.

Sample Foods Cycle 2
Lean Protein
Shellfish (clams, oysters, mussels, scallops, shrimp)
Lean cuts beef (steak, ground beef)
Pork tenderloin, loin roast
Lamb sirloin roast, shanks
Veal

Starches - Complex Carbohydrates - Natural
Grains - 1 portion = 1/2 cup
Brown rice, bulgur, couscous, barley
Cream of wheat, grits, rice (long grain)
Quinoa, oatmeal
Black beans, kidney beans, lima beans, lentils
Soy beans, split peas, navy beans

Starches Vegetables
Potato - 1 portion = 1 medium
Sweet potato
Corn - 1/2 cup
Squash - 1 cup
Breadfruit - 1 cup

Cleansing Vegetables - same as Cycle 1
Fruits - Low- Sugar - same as Cycle 1
Condiments - same as Cycle 1
Fats - same as Cycle 1
Probiotics - same as Cycle 1
Sample Meals 1400-1500 Cal

Day One

Breakfast
Warm lemon water
1/2 cup sugar-free yogurt
1 cup fresh berries
1/2 cup grits with sweetener
Green Tea
Water

Lunch
Grilled pork tenderloin (4 oz)
2 cups mixed greens, tomatoes, carrots, radishes, corn, drizzle low-fat salad dressing
1/2 cup kidney beans
1 mango sliced
Green Tea
Water

Dinner
Sirloin steak (4 oz)
2 cup mixed veggies (broccoli, squash, 2 boiled eggs, eggplant)
Green Tea
Water

Snacks
1/2 cup quinoa
1 cup fresh fruit with 1/2 cup yogurt

Day Two

Breakfast
Warm lemon water
1/2 cup cream of wheat with 2 tbsp wheat germ
1/2 cup raspberries
1 pear sliced

Green Tea
Water

Lunch
1/2 cup sugar-free yogurt
1 cup blueberries
2 cups spinach, carrots, celery, onion, sprouts, tomato,
drizzle fat-free salad dressing
1 boiled egg
Green Tea
Water

Dinner
4 large shrimp
1/2 cup brown rice
2 cups streamed vegetables (carrots, peas, broccoli,
beans, peppers, water chestnuts)
Green Tea
Water

Snack
1/2 cup couscous with 1/2 cup peas/corn
1/2 cup yogurt with a peach

You should be feeling pretty good, getting used to watching what you eat, and how much. The weight should continue to come off during this activation phase. It's important not to overdo it on the starches. There's more lenience with the lean protein and veggies, no cap, except that you stay within the calorie range. Make sure you also continue with your 17 minutes per day of exercise. It doesn't have to be intense, but you do need to be consistent. If you are walking for your exercise, make sure you walk 17 minutes EVERY DAY. If you are hiking or biking, do the same. This is important for your health, results, and it's a part of a balanced lifestyle.

After 17 days in this Active phase or cycle, you'll have graduated to Phase 3.

Phase 3 - Achieve (Day 35-51)

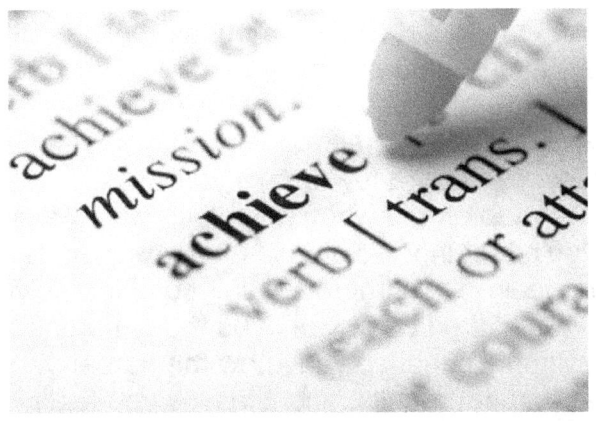

With the Achieve phase of this diet, you are looking to learn healthy eating habits which include portion control, regular eating times, and always making healthy food choices that include foods dense in nutrients, not in calories.

This phase allots you new foods to keep your body and mind guessing, increases the physical up to an hour each day, and still limits your carbs to be in your tummy before 2 each day.

This cycle increases your overall caloric intake and decreases protein; cutting protein consumption by at least a third is ideal. Now don't get too excited here, but now you can enjoy ONE alcoholic beverage per day, a 5 oz class of wine, bottle of beer, or the standard 1.5 oz hard liquor drink. The two full servings of natural starches per day can be eaten before 2 pm, in order to make certain you don't start to plateau in weight loss.

You will keep with the same hydration process of warm lemon water in the morning, Green Tea each meal, and plenty of cool refreshing water.
Calories should be around 1800.

Now is the time to get a touch more serious about exercise. Making sure you get in at least 40-60 minutes of intense aerobic exercise 3-5 times a week. This is a bit of an adjustment, so you need to prepare yourself mentally and persevere. After a few weeks you will start feeling more comfortable, and when combined with the positive results you're seeing; weight loss, energy gain, less aches and pains, and improved self-confidence, you are going to get all fired up to work your body hard in these classes. Simply because you know the harder you work, the faster you get results, and it leaves you feeling fabulous!

Sample Foods Cycle 3
***Lean Protein* - same as Accelerate and Activate cycles.**
Poultry to Add
Canadian bacon
Quail, pheasant, Cornish hen
Low-Fat lunch meat, bacon or sausage

Natural Starches
Whole grain breads
Pumpernickel and rye breads
Whole grain bagels and pitas (serving =1/2 portion)
Small whole grain tortilla
Cereals high in fiber (serving = 1 cup)
All-Bran
Cold cereals that are gluten-free
Granola that's low-fat, low-sugar (serving = 1/2 cup)
Fiber One
Vector

Pasta (serving = 1/2 cup)
Whole grain pasta
Vegetable pasta
High-fiber pasta
Pasta gluten-free

Vegetables - Unlimited
Cleansing veggies same as Accelerate and Activation cycles
Broccoli sprouts, alfalfa, cilantro, chilies, seaweed
Cactus, radishes, rhubarb, Swiss chard, yellow and green beans
Zucchini
Any other veggie you can think of

Fruits - 2 servings each day, 1 piece or 1 cup
All fruits from first 2 cycles
Cherries, bananas, apricots, figs
Papaya, kiwi, pineapple, tangerine
Any fruit

Probiotics
Same as first 2 cycles
Low-fat cheese - 1 serving = 2 ounces
Skim milk - 1 serving = 1 cup
Fat-free cottage cheese or ricotta cheese - 1 serving = 1/2 cup
Sugar-free almond, rice or soy milk for dairy-free - 1 serving = 1 cup

Fats - up to 2 tbsp per day
Avocado - 1/4 fruit
Canola or Walnut oil - 2 tbsp/serving
Light mayonnaise - 2 tbsp/serving
Nuts/seeds - 2 tbsp/serving
Low-fat margarine or dressing - 2 tbsp/serving
Full fat dressing or margarine - 1 tbsp/serving

Snacks under 100 calories
Low-fat Babybell cheese - 2 circles
Low-fat fruit bar or frozen yogurt
Low-fat granola bar
Plain microwave popcorn - 4 cups
Cheese string - 1 portion
Fat-free pudding - 1 cup

Sample Meals

Day One

Breakfast
Warm lemon water
One cup all bran cereal
One cup skim milk
1 cup fresh berries
Green Tea
Water

Lunch
1/2 cup low-fat cottage cheese
Banana
2 cups Romaine, carrots, celery, onions, 1/4 cup avocado, sprouts
1/2 cup couscous
Sliced Mango
Green Tea

Dinner
1 serving grilled sirloin steak
2 cups mixed steamed veggies (green/yellow beans, seaweed, peppers, zucchini)
1 cup low-fat yogurt
Green Tea
Water

Snacks
2 Babybell's
Whole grain granola bar

Day Two

Breakfast
Warm lemon water
4 egg whites
1 cup oatmeal
1 apple sliced
Green Tea

Lunch
Whole grain turkey sandwich (2 slices whole grain bread, 3-4 oz lean turkey, 2 tbsp light mayo, lettuce, tomato, cucumber, onion)
1 oz light cheese
Peach
Green Tea
Water

Dinner
Garden-Cheese salad (2 cups spinach, carrots, cucumber, radishes, carrots, tomato, 1/4 cup sunflower seeds, 1/4 cup fat-free cheese, drizzle fat-free salad dressing)
2 cups steamed veggies of your choice
1 cup vegetable soup
Green Tea
Water

Snacks
Small baked sweet potato
The achieve cycle is all about hitting the mark of what healthy eating and living is all about. By lowering your protein intake and increasing calories, you are deliberately switching gears to help keep your mind and body

focused. The last thing you want to deal with when establishing new habits is a wandering mind.

By keeping starches and fruits before two, you are communicating to your body and internal systems that you want it to keep zapping fat calories, so you can keep losing weight. Don't be shocked if your weight loss slows here because it should. Permanent weight loss has to cycle as the body would naturally, and the 17 Day Diet plays it perfectly.

Adding up to an hour of intense cardio activity 3-5 days a week, is going to ensure your body keeps losing weight. Expect about 5 pounds (give or take) during this cycle. Here, you are getting used to the system. Don't expect perfect, and allow for minor errors. This is the learning phase, fine-tuning will come later.

You should feel really good right now. Happy and proud of your progress, and really getting used to all these positive life changes you have worked so hard to implement! Keep in mind it's always important for you to tailor each step to marry with your preferences and tolerances. If you are unsure of a specific food substitution or otherwise, make sure you ask an expert! Ask and you shall receive. Never give up, keep a healthy perspective, and have patience, all key factors in your success! Up next is Phase 4!

Phase 4 - Arrive (Day 52+)

Consider yourself Arrived! Signifying that you have finally reached your destination. You've established personalized healthy eating habits, and the focus here is learning how to make them stick. The last thing you want to do is regress backwards because you aren't thinking one step ahead of the game.

You feel fabulous right now, having lost the weight you wanted; energy levels are up, your head is clearer, and you are seeing a whole lot of sunshine in your world.

With this phase you are going to keep shocking your system, mind and body, for continuous results. Stopping and starting your metabolism, giving it a little more than less, is going to ensure you don't plateau in the weight loss department, or worse yet start sneaking the weight back on. This phase teaches you how to make sure that just doesn't happen.

By eating in a controlled but healthy fashion for five days, and then allowing for a little bit "free-er" eating for two days, you're rewarding both your mind and body while forcing it to work efficiently and effectively for you.

So for the first 5 days make sure you eat meals that you would have in the first 3 cycles, controlled options. For the 6th and 7th day, you will allow yourself a little bit extra, but no binging, or out of control eating. An extra serving of fruit and veggies here or there, another snack or two, or perhaps an extra portion of whole grain toast with peanut butter is your treat. By now you will understand and appreciate how your body works and how rewarding "more" healthy eating can be.

You will actually get excited about having an extra up of fresh fruit with cottage cheese, or an extra serving of sweet potato fries on occasion. Having a beer, or glass of wine with dinner, is something you can work into your diet in moderation, if that's something you really enjoy. It's also important you still keep up your 60 minutes of intense cardiovascular exercise 3-5 days a week, to help strengthen and tone muscles, increase mobility, decrease aches and pains, burn fat, and give you that "feel good" shot of endorphins that will become addictive.

To ensure you have control here, you should weight yourself on the weekend. If you see your weight isn't where it should be, immediately switch to one of your favorite cycles so you can get right back on track.

This isn't a one stop shop. The 17 Day Diet is a fabulous lifestyle that teaches you how to control your weight and reward yourself. A give-take relationship is all about learning and making adjustments where you see fit. There is no "right" or "wrong" here. It's about gaining knowledge, reasonable perspective, healthy expecta-

tions, and perseverance. The only way you can fail with your new healthy 17 Day Diet lifestyle is to quit.
I'm telling you quitting is NOT an option because YOU ARE WORTH IT!

Strategies to Keep Fat off - Maintenance

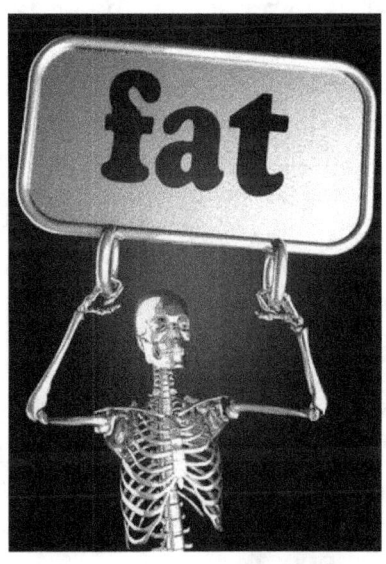

There aren't too many people that don't feel fabulous when they hit their weight loss goal. Agreed? Unfortunately we live in a society where Fad Diets are the norm. A billion dollar industry that fills people full of false hope and extreme strategies to drop fat fast. We want so badly to believe "magic fat blasting wands" really work, we allow our emotion to override logic, and actually convince ourselves that consuming only liquids for the rest of lives is a reasonable expectation. Obviously it isn't, and if you lose 20 pounds fast, by drinking our nutrition, the second you eat "real" food, the fat magically reappears. Leaving you down in the dumps depressed and defeated, with little hope.

You can relate, I'm sure.

I really don't care what "eating strategy" you adopt to lose weight and get healthy. If it's extreme, lacks vital nutrients, doesn't take into consideration the natural rhythm of your body, regular physical exercise, and the ability to keep things interesting and diversified, you are eventually going to derail and plummet over the edge.

* Reasonable expectations have to be set
* All nutrients must be included
* The terms and conditions or "rules" of your new eating strategy has to make sense to YOU
* You need to enjoy this routine of eating, or learn to
* Your new eating strategy has to fit into your version of a healthy lifestyle, one you will learn to make habit, sticking with for life

With The 17 Day Diet, you and create the blueprint of positive nutrition that is going to better you mentally, physically, and emotionally, if that's what you choose. Here are a few key strategies to help you keep your excess weight off for good.

Support System

How come we can so easily disappoint ourselves, often without a second thought? After so many failed weight loss attempts, we seem to get easily discouraged. Throwing in the towel after our first misstep of "chowing" down a tub of triple chocolate ice cream when we're scheduled to be sweating up a storm at the gym.

The guilt unbearable.

Creating a vicious cycle of disaster; extreme dieting and exercising, until we can't stand it anymore, surrendering once again to a pig-out binge that depresses and devastates.

Having someone you trust to hold you accountable is a fantastic support to help keep you on track, particularly in the beginning. This can be a friend or family member, maybe a nutritionist or eating group you've joined. Someone needs to be in place that will inspire you and won't listen to your whining. Rather, they will positively fuel you to reach your weight loss goals, and make sure you stay there. More than one support often works best.

Planning
By planning in everything you do, a road is created that leads to success. Planning is productive, and increases the chances you're going to reach your goal. A house can't be built without planning. A Christmas dinner isn't going to run smoothly without a master plan of attack.

The same goes with the 17 Day Diet. If you don't plan out and know what you're going to eat and when, BEFORE it's time to eat, there's going to be trouble. This could leave you starving and more willing to snack, when you're trying to figure out what to make. Worse yet, you may grab something you shouldn't be eating just because you can't be bothered to run to the grocery store to get food. I think you see where I'm headed here.

Plan your meals at least 2-3 days in a row, so that when your tummy tells it's time to eat, you don't have to use your brain cells to figure out what. If you are really organized and can buy all your groceries on Sunday for the week, that's even better.

Measuring Routinely
As humans, we need to see and measure progress as incentive to keep on going. If you are a runner, you will time yourself to see if you get faster with the adjustments you've made in your training. A prime example of a measuring tool.

When it comes to losing weight and getting healthy, there are lots of tools people use to measure. Some people go by how their clothes fit. If they're starting to get snug, action needs to be taken. Others may tune into their body, and go by how they are feeling.

The most accurate and level way to keep on track with your hard-earned weight loss, is to step on the scale periodically. This is the quickest route to making sure you're maintaining your weight and lifestyle changes.

Notice - Weighing yourself too often isn't a good thing, because your body needs time to shed fat and work through the cycle. Getting a reading once a week on the weekend is plenty. Remembering the importance of wearing the same clothes, at the same time of day, so you get a little more accurate reading. In your birthday suit really is the best, but I'll leave that one up to you. Taking body fat measurements also works. Just make sure you are using the tape measure accurately. This in combination with the scale is best. Once every two weeks is plenty.

Journals also work great, where you record your days in detail. Examples entries would be: How you were feeling? What you ate? The pounds lost, and so forth. This gives you something concrete to look back on whenever you like to remind you of just how far you've come, how much progress you've made.

By making a habit of recording your progress and even your setbacks, you're much more likely to hold yourself accountable to you.

Use Your Crystal Ball
It's important to troubleshoot where you can. Perhaps you have some people you hang out with that choose to

eat unhealthy, and won't take no for an answer. Maybe you need to steer clear of them while you're getting yourself established with the 17 Day Diet?

You may be programmed to always have snacks at the Saturday afternoon show. Improvise, by making sure you eat before you go. Maybe you can work in 4 cups of your own popcorn for a snack, and can treat yourself to a diet Green Tea, opting for some sugar-less gum instead of chips and candy during the show? Theater popcorn is very bad for you, so just don't make it an option. Where there's a will there's a way, and if you use your crystal ball you're going to be successful.

Accept you're Human
So what? You had a couple squares at the party, or ended up having a serving of mashed potatoes at 6pm. Let it go. You're human and life happens. The important factor here is that you realize what you did, and just need to tighten up the strings a little, and get right back on track. You will find the further along you get on the 17 Day Diet the more forgiving your body will be.

A great method of counteracting any damage done with an eating mistake, is to throw in some extra exercise. Remembering this is all about give and take. So you had 3 light beers at a friend's party when you should have had just one? No worries! That's about 200 extra calories. By adding 30 minutes extra of moderate biking, you will level the playing field. This sort of thinking is invaluable when looking to maintain your gains.

This strategy can be executed by cutting back a little on each of your meals after you've had a few too many calories. Keeping in mind, if you lower your calories too much, this will force your body to battle you in fat loss.

Increase Activity Outside of Eating

Remember, out of sight, out of mind. By keeping yourself busy with hobbies and other interests, you're not going to me so focused on good. If you don't have any hobbies get some. Think of things you've always wanted to try and get to it! Maybe you want to learn how to paint, roller-skate, bowl, or play bingo. The idea here, is to get more involved and interested in all that life has to offer, to fill the food void you may have been focused on at one time. Change is good.

Diversify

This is the spice of life. Diversity keeps things exciting, and when it comes to maintaining weight loss, diversity is king! Mixing up the foods you are eating and the exercise you are doing, is going to push your body to burn more calories and keep yourself from slipping into boredom. Excitement is the spice of life, effective exercising and weight loss.

If you catch yourself getting a little too much into routine, that's your cue to make a few minor adjustments. This can be as simple as picking up the pace in your walk for five minutes, and then back down to normal for the re-mainder.

Reward Yourself

We work for reward in everything, and if it's missing, veering off course is more likely to become reality. If you lose 15 pounds after Phase 1, you should reward your-self for your efforts. Treat yourself to a new pair of pants, a specialty Green Tea at the new coffee shop, or maybe you're a "shoe-a-holic," and with each goal a new pair of shoes goes into your closet?

It doesn't matter how big or small your reward, just make sure you do recognize and reward your efforts regularly. That's incentive to move forward full speed ahead.

My Thinking . . .
Having a maintenance plan in place is critical with the 17 Day Diet, or any other newly established eating strategy for that matter. Why would you want to risk gaining all your fat back, and falling back into your old and un-healthy eating? Prevention is the key and having a maintenance plan in place will remind you of all the posi-tive health changes you are making.
Your health and wellness is too important to ignore, and maintenance is a must for long-term success.

Neat Food Factoids

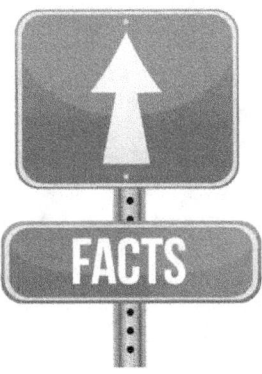

Food is something we all have in common. Here are some weird and interesting food facts that may be news to you.

- Peanuts are technically legumes and not nuts. They're also used to make dynamite!
- It may not surprise you that Coke was originally green.
- Ketchup was sold in the early 1800s as medicine.
- Coconut water can be used as blood plasma in emergencies because it's sterile and has a compatible PH.
- The first recorded soup was hippopotamus.
- Vinegar has the ability to melt pearls.
- Carrots were initially grown for "Karoto" medicine, by the ancient Greeks.
- Worcestershire sauce is made from anchovies dissolved in vinegar.
- Avocados are poisonous to birds, and contain the most protein of any fruit.
- Spam will last for eternity in an unopened can.
- Grapes explode in the microwave. It's true!

- Cherries are a part of the rose family.
- Bananas technically aren't a fruit, they're an herb.
- If you bounce a cranberry high, it's ripe to eat.
- Ears of corn will always have an even number of rows.
- The darker the pumpkin shell, the longer it lasts

My Thoughts . . .
This was just a few neat food facts to add to your
knowledge base. Information is knowledge and
knowledge is power. Open your thoughts to search for
gain.

The "Mental" of Dieting

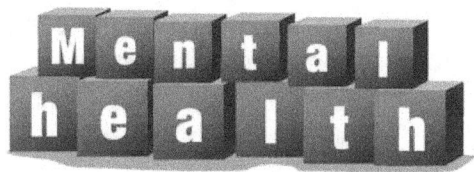

Having a positive mental attitude in anything is important. When it comes to dieting and the 17 Day Diet, a positive attitude will set you up for success. Positive thinking is what carries you through those "tough" days, where you just can't seem to muster up the energy you'd like. Those times where you happen to be feeling down or blue, things just aren't going as planned. This is where conscious positive mental thinking will make the world of difference.

It's learned and takes time, patience, and commitment. Anyone can start a diet plan and be all excited initially. This wears off fast, and having positive thinking is only going to help you stick with it faithfully for the long haul. I daresay the most important component of a diet plan is a positive mindset.

Your Mental and the 17 Day Diet Plan
The mind is a powerful thing, and if you think it, you can do it. Your thoughts are what dictate your actions, and

often just putting random things into your head are the beginnings of a new reality to be. Think of the "thought" as the seed in the garden. Without the seed, you will never have a beautiful flower. Without committing to the healthy eating strategies of the 17 Day Diet with a positive mental attitude, you'll have a tough time sticking with it for life.

Positive thinking means you aren't going to quit, and you'll be able to overcome any barriers that pop up, particularly the emotional and truly powerful ones of self-doubt.

Positive Mental Thinking will keep you on Track
If you program your head to be positive, you are always going to set supports to ensure your weight loss success. Maybe there's a cute little black dress you really want to fit into? Your positive mental thinking will remind you, this is the first thing you're going to purchase WHEN you drop the weight.

Maybe you are running for your cardio exercise in Phase 3, and really find the last 15 minutes challenging. Your positive thinking will override this negativity, reminding you there's a huge ice cold bottle of lemon water waiting for you when you finish.

A positive head is a focused head, one that will create an environment where you are inevitably going to succeed.

Helps Relate Positive to Dieting
We are conditioned to associate "dieting" with negative. Deprivation, no energy, starvation, and all sorts of other depressing thoughts naturally pop up when you hear the word diet.

This is all in our head; a matter of perception, and if you consciously choose to see the good in things, you will. Your reality is what you make it. If you tell your mind that dieting is not a negative thing, and that it's all about making positive changes that will better you and your life, you WILL believe it and it WILL happen. All you've got to do is focus on it and believe.

Ensures you Surpass Emotional Hurdles
Emotional eating is the causal factor for many overweight people. Many don't even realize they are eating when they aren't even hungry. They've created a habit to grab chips when they are depressed after getting dumped. Or if as emotional eater has a bad day at work, an ice cream on the way home acts as short-term therapy. Sure, it may boost your spirits temporarily, with a fast injection of sugar into your system. Sadly, it doesn't last, and then you've created a depressed feeling, and the guilt of unhealthy eating to deal with.

Studies show happier people are less depressed, and have a decreased likelihood of eating because of their emotions, or in the least, learning how to recognize the triggers and control them. This is the key to losing weight, and sticking to your 17 Day Diet weight loss strategy.

My Thoughts . . .
When you are thinking in a positive light, you are focused on sunshine. Success is something you strive towards, rather than make excuses to never get there. With a little time and patience, and whole lot of persistence, you will make positive thinking a staple for you, and this is going to push you though to the finish line of each and every one of your weight loss and life goals.

Physical and Dieting

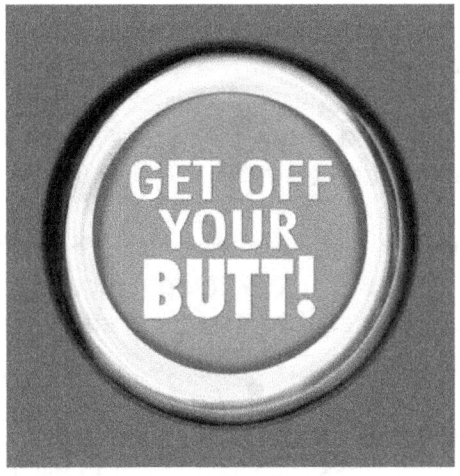

Your body was built to be physical EVERY DAY. It's programmed in your genes, and when you deny your body by lazing on the couch, and driving when you could be walking, you are only harming your health.

Each of your internal systems that control your emotional, physical, and mental, are reliant on an intricately timed group of systems. These systems run more efficiently and effectively with regular exercise. "You snooze - you lose," when it comes to moving your body. If you choose not to exercise, you'll lose mobility and agility, clear thinking and energy, aches and pains will become your focus, and routine daily activities will require pain and huge effort.

Establishing healthy and sensible eating with the 17 Day Diet, combined with regular physical exercise, is exactly what will set you up for permanent weight loss, and a long and healthy life.

Other exercise benefits are:

Decrease Risk of Serious Disease - Exercising regularly as the 17 Day Diet encourages, will help lower your chances of developing serious disease. Heart disease, stroke, diabetes, and various cancers, are a few common ailments exercise can deter.

Lowers Blood Pressure - A risk factor of cardiovascular disease and stroke is high blood pressure. Regular exercise lowers blood pressure and cholesterol naturally.

Reduction of Aches and Pains - Many of us just assume aches and pains are "normal." By taking care of your body with regular physical exercise, you will immediately notice many of your "usual "aches and pains will magically disappear.

Lower Back Pain - Routine physical exercise will naturally strengthen back muscles, improve circulation, release "feel good" hormones, and help to alleviate lower back pain without harmful medications. If you can provide pain relief naturally, and prevent progression, why wouldn't you?

Endorphin Release - Exercise that gets your heart rate up naturally, releases endorphins (hormones), which boost your spirits long after you've finished exercising. These chemicals help to mask pain, and leave you feeling energetic and positive. Many, including me, believe these chemicals are addictive, and that's all good.

Triggers Metabolic Boost - Of course a highlight of exercise is boosting the calories burned, and this means if you are eating the right foods, fat loss will be increased. Regular physical exercise with smart eating, like the 17 Day Diet, is going to speed up the rate in which you lose fat AND boost your positive perspective, a double win for you.

* Improves Mobility - Routine physical exercise naturally improves motility and leaves you mobile longer. If you are moving around more, you will be "able" to do this longer. If you are stuck in a chair day after day without exercise, eventually you will lose the ability to walk or move without pain. It's your choice to get moving or else!

My Thoughts . . .
The 17 Day Diet includes regular physical activity from the start. It's important to begin slow and work your way up, listen to your body, and always check with your doctor before beginning just to be safe.

Exercising regularly improves you mentally, physically, emotionally, and socially, all positively. Keeping it diverse and exciting will starve off boredom, and force your body to give you results fast, never hitting a plateau and always reaching your weight loss goals sooner, not later. Ideally, 45 minutes to an hour, 3-5 days a week works. It's important for you to find what fits for you, committing to work hard to make it habit.

Final Words

As mentioned previous, there is no "perfect" diet or exercise program. There's always room for improvement, and you need to make the adjustments necessary in each to make them "fit" your tolerances and preferences.

What works for your best friend, may not work for you, and that's okay. You owe it to yourself to use the 17 Day Diet and make it work for you. Tweak it where you need to, and find your rhythm. This diet is the fastest route for you to lose fat, gain energy, increase motility and agility, deter disease, and make better of the symptoms you might be suffering from any chronic conditions.

The 17 Day Diet is going to teach you a sensible strategy to giving your body the right amount of vitamins and minerals to run optimally, while allowing you to control your weight loss. Fast and effective is what the 17 Day Diet is. All that's left now is for you to experience it!

Last Thoughts…

*THANK-YOU for reading my masterpiece. I hope you learned a little something, or at least got a few smiles.

*I would appreciate a millisecond or three of your time for a quick review, to help me build my masterful book empire higher.

*Whatever you do,don't forget to smile, and of course, check out my website for more of my e-Book masterpieces!

Visit my website at: flawlesscreatvewriting.com

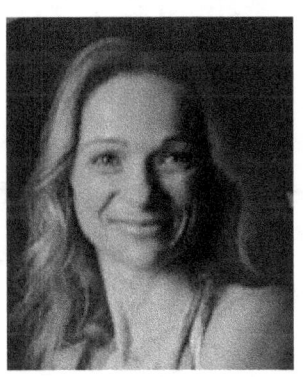

Cathy☺

Disclaimer

www.ingramcontent.com/pod-product-compliance
Lightning Source LLC
Chambersburg PA
CBHW060219290526
45789CB00003B/1323